MANAGING AILMENTS

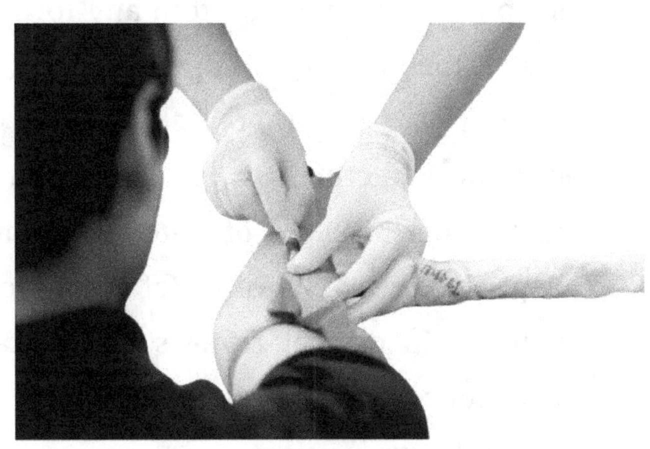

*Optimizing Wellness:
Effective Strategies For
Managing Ailments*

Bridget Sisan

Table of contents

Introduction

In a quaint town nestled between rolling hills, lived Lily, a woman burdened by chronic ailments. Frustrated with traditional treatments, she stumbled upon an old bookstore and found a mysterious, leather-bound book titled "Healing Pages." Intrigued, Lily delved into the ancient wisdom within its pages. The book unfolded a tapestry of holistic approaches, blending herbs, mindfulness, and dietary changes. As she absorbed the knowledge, Lily started implementing these practices into her daily life.

Over weeks, subtle shifts occurred. Lily's chronic pain began to wane, her energy levels surged, and a newfound vitality blossomed. The book became her guide, offering solace and empowerment. Lily shared her journey with the town, and soon others, inspired by her success, embraced the healing wisdom within "Healing Pages." The bookstore transformed into a hub of communal support, as people exchanged insights and experiences. Lily's story echoed through the town, sparking a ripple effect of wellness. The once-ailing community flourished, not only physically but also spiritually.

As seasons changed, the bookstore became a symbol of hope and transformation. Lily, now vibrant and healthy, continued to explore the pages of "Healing Pages," discovering new facets of well-being. The town, once resigned to ailments, bloomed into a haven of vitality, all thanks to the power of a book and the courage of one woman to embrace its teachings.

Managing ailments is a multifaceted approach that encompasses various strategies to promote well-being and alleviate health challenges. Ailments, ranging from minor discomforts to chronic conditions, necessitate careful attention and proactive measures to enhance overall quality of life. This comprehensive process involves a combination of preventive measures, lifestyle adjustments, medical interventions, and holistic approaches. By understanding the underlying factors contributing to ailments and adopting a tailored management plan, individuals can strive to mitigate symptoms, improve resilience, and foster long-term health and vitality. This introduction sets the stage for exploring the diverse facets of ailment management, emphasizing the importance of a holistic and personalized approach to address the complexities of health and wellness.

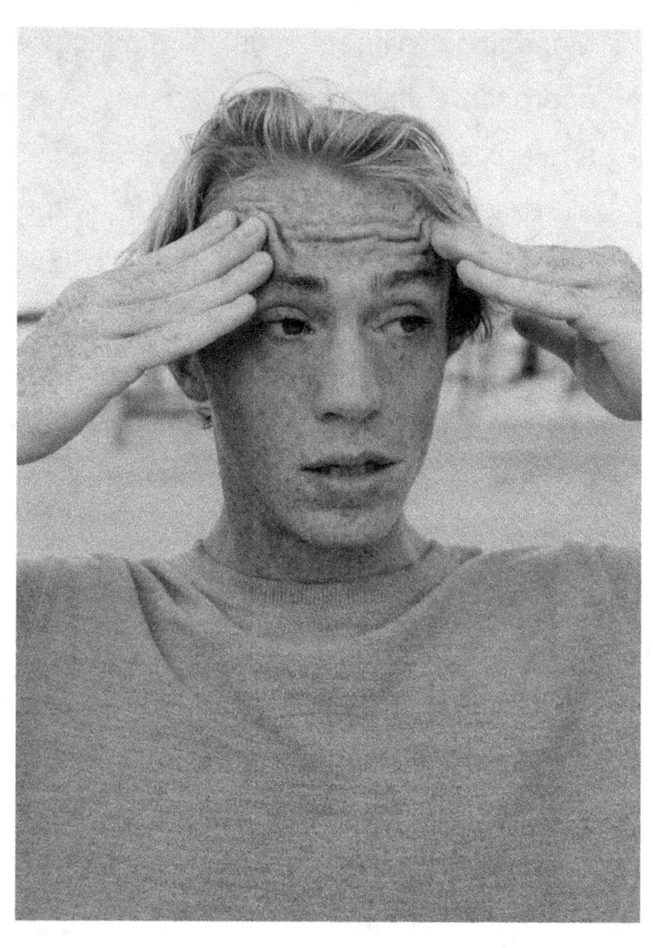

Chapter 1. Purpose of Ailment Management

Ailment management serves the crucial purpose of enhancing the quality of life for individuals dealing with health challenges. This comprehensive approach involves the coordinated efforts of healthcare professionals, patients, and their support networks to mitigate the impact of ailments. The key objectives include:

1. **Symptom Control:** Ailment management aims to alleviate and control symptoms effectively. This involves the use of medications, therapies, and lifestyle adjustments tailored to the specific ailment,

providing relief and improving overall well-being.

2.   Prevention   of   Complications: Managing ailments helps prevent the development of complications. Through regular monitoring and proactive interventions, healthcare professionals can identify potential risks and implement strategies to minimize their impact on the individual's health.

3. **Optimizing Functionality**: The goal is to enable individuals to maintain or regain optimal functionality despite their ailment. This may involve physical rehabilitation, occupational therapy, and other interventions aimed at improving daily activities and independence.

4. **Enhancing Adherence to Treatmen**t: Effective ailment management involves promoting patient adherence to prescribed treatments. Education, counseling, and support services play a crucial role in ensuring that individuals understand and follow their treatment plans, leading to better health outcomes.

5. Improving Quality of Life: Ailment management seeks to enhance the overall quality of life for individuals by addressing not only physical symptoms but also emotional and social aspects. Psychosocial support, mental health interventions, and community involvement contribute to a holistic approach to well-being.

6. Patient Empowerment: Empowering patients with knowledge and skills to actively participate in their own care is a fundamental aspect of ailment management. This includes education about their condition, self-care practices, and strategies to cope with challenges.

7. Resource Optimization: Ailment management aims to optimize healthcare resources by preventing unnecessary hospitalizations and emergency room visits.

This is achieved through proactive monitoring, early intervention, and effective outpatient care.

8. Long-term Health Maintenance: Ailment management is often a lifelong process for chronic conditions. It involves creating sustainable strategies to maintain health over the long term, emphasizing preventative measures and ongoing support.

9. Cost-Efficiency: Proactive ailment management can contribute to cost savings in the healthcare system by reducing the need for emergency interventions and expensive treatments. Preventing complications and hospitalizations can result in more efficient resource utilization.

In conclusion, ailment management is a multifaceted approach aimed at improving the lives of individuals facing health challenges. By addressing symptoms, preventing complications, empowering patients, and optimizing resources, this comprehensive strategy seeks to promote not just the absence of disease but the highest possible level of physical, mental, and social well-being.

Importance of Early Intervention

Early intervention plays a pivotal role in managing ailments across various medical conditions. Timely identification and intervention significantly contribute to improved outcomes, reduced severity of symptoms, and enhanced overall well-being.

One crucial aspect of early intervention is the ability to identify potential health issues at their incipient stages. Regular health screenings and check-ups enable healthcare professionals to detect abnormalities or risk factors before they escalate into serious ailments. This proactive approach allows for prompt diagnosis and implementation of appropriate interventions, minimizing the impact on an individual's health.

In many cases, early intervention proves crucial in preventing the progression of diseases. By addressing health concerns at an early stage, healthcare providers can implement targeted treatments, lifestyle modifications, or preventive measures. This not only helps in managing the ailment effectively but also reduces the likelihood of complications and long-term health issues.

For developmental conditions and disorders, such as autism or learning disabilities, early intervention is particularly vital. During the early stages of a child's life, their brain undergoes rapid development, and interventions aimed at promoting healthy development can have a profound impact. Early identification and intervention in developmental delays can lead to improved cognitive, social, and emotional outcomes.

In the context of chronic diseases, early intervention can often slow down or even halt the progression of the ailment. For conditions like diabetes or hypertension, prompt management through lifestyle changes, medication, or other interventions can prevent complications such as cardiovascular diseases, kidney damage, or nerve problems.

Beyond individual health, early intervention also plays a crucial role in public health initiatives. Swift responses to emerging infectious diseases, for example, can help contain outbreaks and prevent widespread transmission. Vaccination programs, early detection of contagious diseases, and effective public health measures contribute to the overall well-being of communities.

Additionally, early intervention has economic implications. The cost of managing a health condition tends to increase as it progresses. By addressing ailments at an early stage, healthcare systems can potentially reduce the financial burden associated with prolonged treatments, hospitalizations, and rehabilitation.

In conclusion, the importance of early intervention in managing ailments cannot be overstated. Whether in preventing the progression of chronic diseases, promoting healthy development in children, or responding to emerging health threats, early identification and timely intervention are fundamental to achieving positive health outcomes for individuals and communities alike.

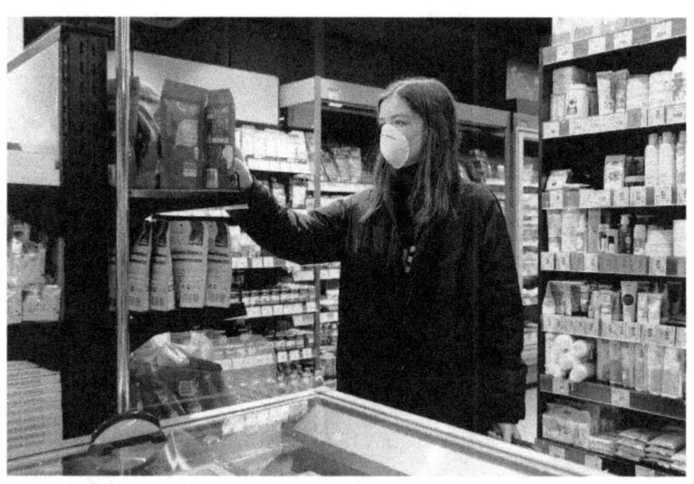

Chapter 2. Understanding Ailments

Understanding ailments is crucial for maintaining overall well-being. Ailments refer to various health conditions or disorders that affect the normal functioning of the body. They can range from minor, temporary discomforts to chronic, life-altering conditions. Here's a comprehensive guide to understanding ailments.

1. Definition of Ailments:

Ailments encompass a broad spectrum of health issues, including physical, mental, and emotional disturbances. They can affect any part of the body and may result from various factors such as genetics, lifestyle, environmental influences, or infectious agents.

2. Types of Ailments:

- **Acute Ailments:** These are short-term conditions that often have a sudden onset, like the common cold or a sprained ankle.

- **Chronic Ailments:** These are long-lasting conditions, such as diabetes, hypertension, or arthritis, requiring ongoing management and care.

- **Infectious Ailments:** Caused by pathogens like bacteria, viruses, fungi, or parasites, examples include influenza, tuberculosis, and malaria.

- **Mental Health Ailments:** Conditions affecting mental well-being, like depression, anxiety disorders, or schizophrenia.

3. Causes of Ailments:

- **Genetic Factors:** Some ailments have a hereditary component, making individuals more susceptible if there's a family history.

- **Environmental Factors:** Exposure to pollutants, toxins, or a lack of essential nutrients can contribute to ailment development.

Lifestyle Choices: Poor diet, lack of exercise, smoking, excessive alcohol consumption, and stress can increase the risk of various ailments.

4. Symptoms and Diagnosis:

- Recognizing symptoms is crucial for early detection. Symptoms vary widely depending on the ailment but may include pain, fatigue, fever, changes in appetite, or mood swings.
- Diagnosis often involves medical tests, imaging, and physical examinations conducted by healthcare professionals.

5. Prevention and Management:

- **Healthy Lifestyle:** Adopting a balanced diet, regular exercise, adequate sleep, and stress management can prevent many ailments.

- **Vaccinations:** Immunizations help prevent infectious ailments and contribute to public health.
- **Regular Check-ups:** Routine medical check-ups enable early detection and intervention, enhancing the chances of successful management.

6. Treatment Approaches:

- **Medication:** Prescription or over-the-counter drugs are often used to manage symptoms or treat the underlying causes of ailments.
- **Therapies:** Physical therapy, psychotherapy, and other specialized interventions may be recommended for specific ailments.
- **Surgery:** In some cases, surgical procedures are necessary to address ailments, especially those affecting organs or tissues.

7. Emotional and Social Impact:

- Ailments can have profound emotional and social consequences. Individuals may experience stigma, isolation, or changes in relationships.
- Support from family, friends, and mental health professionals is crucial in coping with the emotional challenges associated with ailments.

8. Advancements in Ailment Research:

- Ongoing scientific research and medical advancements contribute to better understanding ailments, leading to improved prevention, diagnosis, and treatment options.

In conclusion, understanding ailments involves recognizing their diverse nature, addressing risk factors, and adopting proactive health measures. A holistic approach, considering both physical and mental well-being, is essential for maintaining a healthy and fulfilling life. Regular healthcare check-ups, healthy lifestyle choices, and staying informed about emerging research contribute to a proactive approach in dealing with ailments.

Common Ailments and Their Causes

Common ailments and their causes vary widely, but understanding them is crucial for effective management. Respiratory issues, like colds, often result from viral infections, while allergies stem from hypersensitivity to allergens. Digestive problems, such as indigestion, can be triggered by overeating or consuming spicy foods. Musculoskeletal pain may arise from poor posture or overexertion. poor nutrition and lack of exercise.

Chronic conditions, like hypertension, often link to lifestyle factors such as diet and stress. Skin ailments, such as acne, may be influenced by hormonal imbalances and skincare habits. Mental health issues, like anxiety, can be caused by a combination of genetic, environmental, and psychological factors.

Managing ailments involves adopting a balanced lifestyle, seeking medical advice when needed, taking prescribed medications, and incorporating preventive measures such as vaccination and regular health check-ups.

Recognizing Symptoms

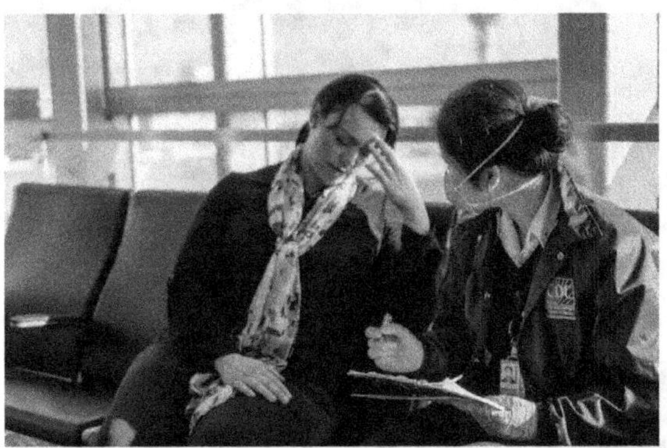

Recognizing symptoms is crucial for managing ailments effectively. Regularly monitor changes in your body, such as unusual pain, fatigue, or persistent discomfort. Consult healthcare professionals promptly for accurate diagnosis and early intervention, as early detection often leads to better outcomes. Keep a health journal to track symptoms, triggers, and patterns, aiding healthcare providers in comprehensive assessments. Prioritize open communication with your healthcare team to ensure personalized and timely care, optimizing your overall well-being

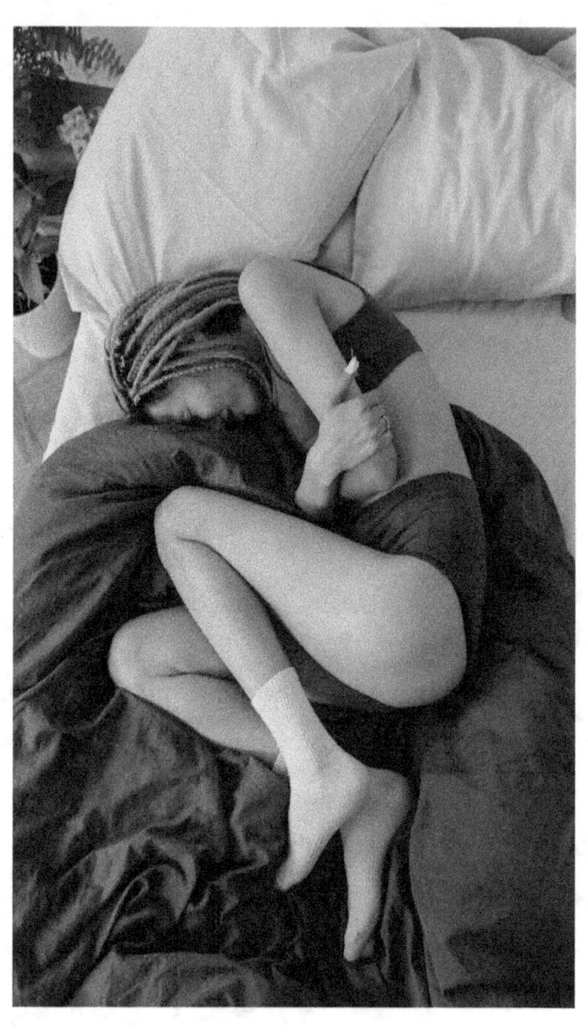

Chapter 3. Seeking Professional Help

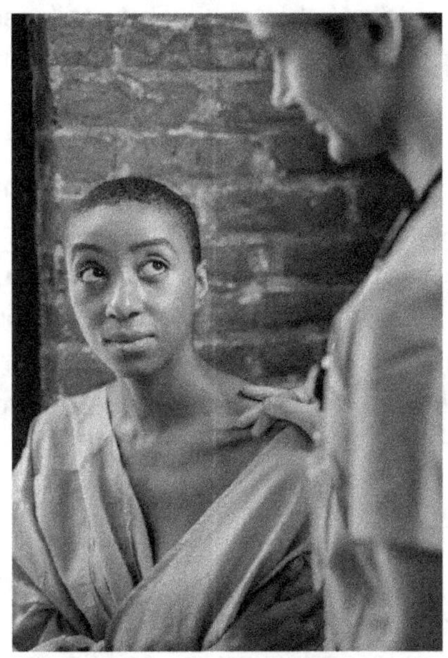

Seeking professional help in managing ailments is crucial for both physical and mental well-being. Whether it's a physical illness or a mental health issue, consulting healthcare professionals ensures accurate diagnosis and effective treatment plans. Doctors, therapists, and specialists possess the expertise to assess symptoms, recommend appropriate interventions, and guide patients toward recovery.

Ignoring or self-diagnosing ailments can lead to complications and prolonged suffering. Professional healthcare providers offer personalized care, considering individual needs and medical history. This tailored approach enhances the likelihood of successful outcomes and improved quality of life.

In the realm of mental health, therapists and counselors provide essential support for issues like anxiety, depression, and stress. They offer a safe space to explore emotions, develop coping mechanisms, and foster resilience. Seeking professional help is a proactive step towards addressing mental health challenges and building a foundation for long-term well-being.

Remember, taking charge of your health includes recognizing when it's time to consult professionals who can provide the necessary expertise and support for managing ailments effectively.

Choosing the Right Healthcare Provider

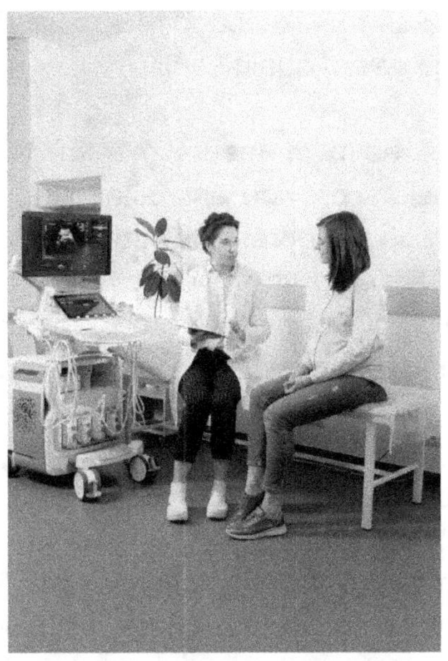

Seeking professional help in managing ailments is crucial for both physical and mental well-being. Whether it's a physical illness or a mental health issue, consulting healthcare professionals ensures accurate diagnosis and effective treatment plans. Doctors, therapists, and specialists possess the expertise to assess symptoms, recommend appropriate interventions, and guide patients toward recovery.

Ignoring or self-diagnosing ailments can lead to complications and prolonged suffering. Professional healthcare providers offer personalized care, considering individual needs and medical history. This tailored approach enhances the likelihood of successful outcomes and improved quality of life.

In the realm of mental health, therapists and counselors provide essential support for issues like anxiety, depression, and stress. They offer a safe space to explore emotions, develop coping mechanisms, and foster resilience. Seeking professional help is a proactive step towards addressing mental health challenges and building a foundation for long-term well-being.

Remember, taking charge of your health includes recognizing when it's time to consult professionals who can provide the necessary expertise and support for managing ailments effectively.

Scheduling Regular Check-ups

Regular checkups are crucial for managing ailments effectively. Schedule routine appointments with your healthcare provider to monitor your health, discuss any concerns, and adjust your treatment plan if needed. Consistent checkups can help detect potential issues early, ensuring timely intervention and improving overall health outcomes.

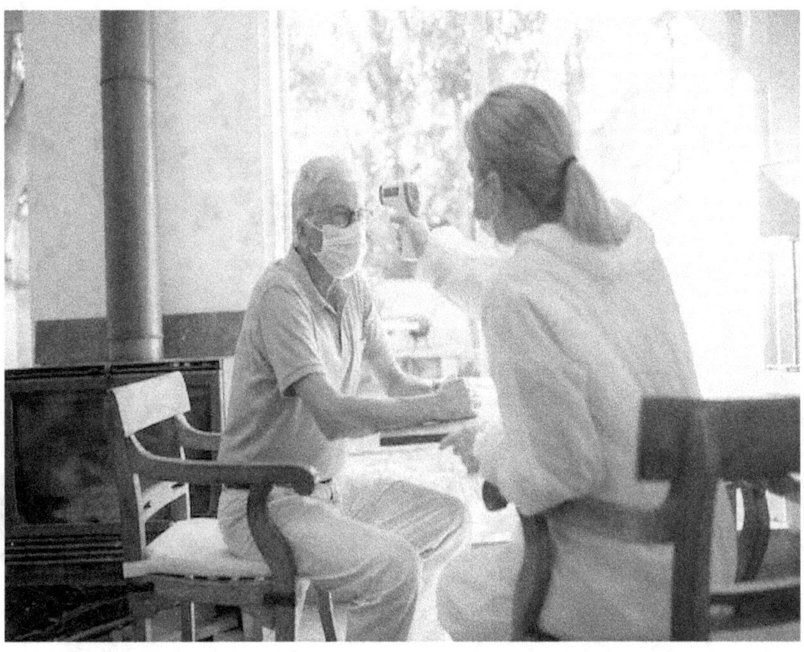

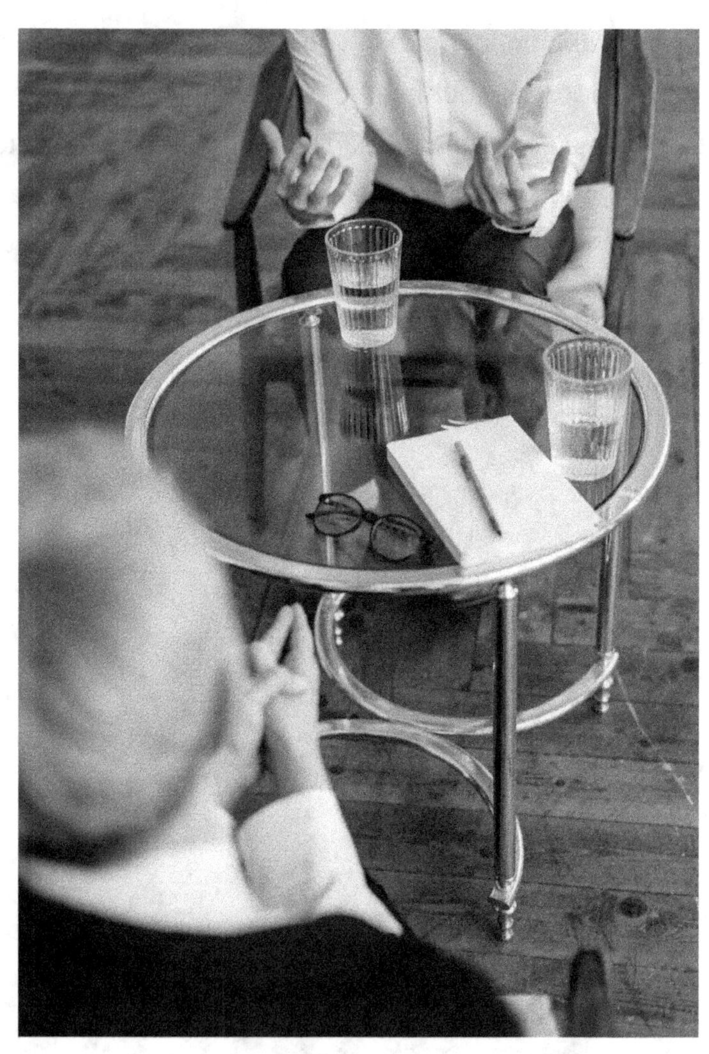

Chapter 4.
Self-Assessment and Monitoring

Self-assessment and monitoring play crucial roles in managing ailments, empowering individuals to take an active role in their health. This proactive approach involves regular evaluation of one's physical and mental well-being, aiding in the early detection of potential issues and fostering a more personalized healthcare strategy.

1. Understanding Self-Assessment:
- Self-assessment involves evaluating various aspects of one's health, including physical, emotional, and lifestyle factors.
- It begins with awareness of symptoms, tracking changes in health, and recognizing patterns over time.

2. Physical Health Monitoring:

- Regularly measure vital signs like blood pressure, heart rate, and temperature.
- Keep track of weight, as fluctuations may indicate underlying issues.
- Monitor specific symptoms related to the ailment, noting any variations.

3. Emotional and Mental Well-being:
- Recognize and address changes in mood, stress levels, or sleep patterns.
- Practice mindfulness and stress management techniques to promote mental health.
- Seek professional help if experiencing persistent emotional challenges.

4. Lifestyle Evaluation:
- Assess daily habits, including diet, exercise, and sleep patterns.
- Identify triggers or factors exacerbating the ailment.
- Make informed adjustments to lifestyle choices for improved overall well-being.

5. Utilizing Health Journals:
- Maintain a health journal to record symptoms, activities, and noteworthy events.
- Document medication schedules and any side effects experienced.

- Provide a comprehensive overview for healthcare professionals during consultations.

6. Technology-Assisted Monitoring:
- Leverage health apps and wearable devices for real-time tracking.
- Set reminders for medication, appointments, and health-related tasks.
- Share collected data with healthcare providers for more informed decision-making.

7. Establishing Baselines:
- Establish baseline measurements for key health indicators.
- Regularly compare current values to baseline data to identify deviations.
- Recognize normal fluctuations and alarming trends.

8. Regular Check-ins with Healthcare Professionals:
- Make time for routine examinations and appointments with medical professionals.
- Share self-assessment findings and collaborate on adjustments to the care plan.
- Stay informed about new treatment options and advancements in managing the ailment.

9. Empowering Patient Advocacy:
- Motivate patients to take an active role in their medical care.
- Develop a strong partnership with healthcare providers, fostering open communication.
- Advocate for personalized treatment plans based on individual self-assessment and monitoring results.

10. Importance of Timely Intervention:
- Early detection through self-assessment allows for timely intervention.
- Prompt adjustments to treatment plans can prevent complications and improve outcomes.
- Empower individuals to be proactive in managing their health for a higher quality of life.

In conclusion, self-assessment and monitoring are integral components of effective ailment management, promoting a holistic approach to health. By actively participating in their well-being, individuals can make informed decisions, collaborate with healthcare professionals, and enhance the overall effectiveness of their treatment plans.

Tracking Symptoms

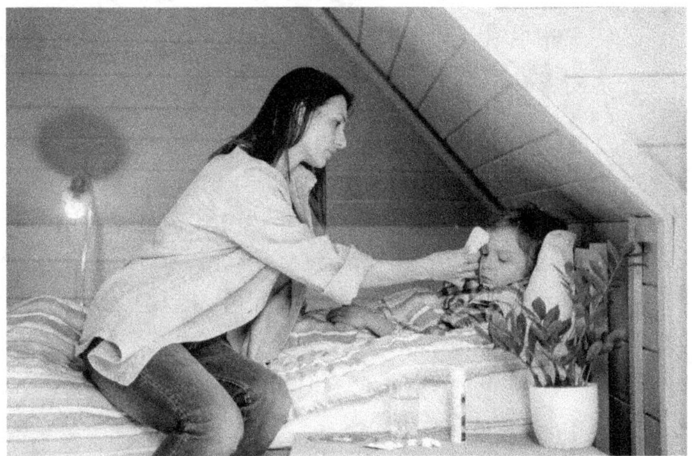

Monitoring symptoms is crucial for managing ailments effectively. Regular tracking allows individuals and their healthcare providers to identify patterns, assess treatment efficacy, and make informed decisions. Here's a guide on tracking symptoms for better ailment management:

1. Keep a Symptom Journal:

Start by maintaining a symptom journal. Record the date, time, and severity of each symptom. Include details like duration, triggers, and any activities or foods that might influence the symptoms.

2. Use Tracking Apps:

Leverage technology by using symptom tracking apps. These apps often provide user-friendly interfaces, reminders, and the ability to generate reports. Popular apps include Symple, Healthily, or customized apps specific to certain ailments.

3. Identify Triggers:

Pay attention to potential triggers. Whether it's specific foods, environmental factors, stress, or sleep patterns, understanding triggers can help modify behavior and lifestyle to alleviate symptoms.

4. Scale Symptoms:

Use a scale to measure the intensity of symptoms. This can be a numerical scale or descriptive terms like mild, moderate, or severe. Consistency in rating helps in establishing trends over time.

5. Track Medication and Treatments:

Record details about medications, dosages, and treatments. Note any side effects experienced. This information aids healthcare professionals in adjusting or changing the treatment plan if necessary.

6. Regular Check-ins with Healthcare Providers:

Share your symptom tracking records during appointments. This provides healthcare providers with valuable insights into your condition, enabling them to make more informed decisions about your care.

7. Set Goals and Monitor Progress:

Establish realistic goals for symptom management. Regularly review your progress and adjust goals as needed. This helps in staying motivated and actively engaged in the management process.

8. Educate Yourself:

Stay informed about your ailment and symptoms. Understanding the condition empowers you to identify relevant symptoms and communicate effectively with healthcare professionals.

9. Consider Biometric Tracking:

For certain ailments, tracking biometrics like blood pressure, heart rate, or blood glucose levels can provide additional insights. Use dedicated devices or integrate with smartphones for seamless tracking.

10. Share with Support Network:

If comfortable, share your symptom tracking information with a trusted support network. This can be beneficial for emotional support and practical assistance when needed.

Remember, effective symptom tracking is a collaborative effort between individuals and healthcare providers. Consistent and accurate records enhance the overall management of ailments, contributing to improved quality of life.

Utilizing Health Apps and Tools

Health apps and tools play a crucial role in managing ailments by providing accessible resources for monitoring, tracking, and improving overall well-being. These tools can assist in medication adherence, symptom tracking, and lifestyle adjustments, offering personalized insights to users.

By integrating health apps into daily routines, individuals can actively manage chronic conditions such as diabetes, hypertension, or mental health issues. These apps often feature reminders for medication schedules, tools for monitoring vital signs, and educational resources to empower users with relevant information about their conditions.

Moreover, fitness and nutrition apps contribute to holistic ailment management by promoting healthy habits. They offer exercise routines tailored to specific conditions and dietary guidance to support overall wellness. Wearable devices further enhance this experience by continuously collecting real-time data, allowing for a more comprehensive understanding of one's health status.

The data generated by these apps can be shared with healthcare professionals, enabling more informed and collaborative decision-making. Telemedicine platforms also leverage health apps to facilitate remote consultations, making healthcare more accessible and efficient.

In summary, the integration of health apps and tools into daily life empowers individuals to actively manage their ailments, fostering a proactive and informed approach to healthcare.

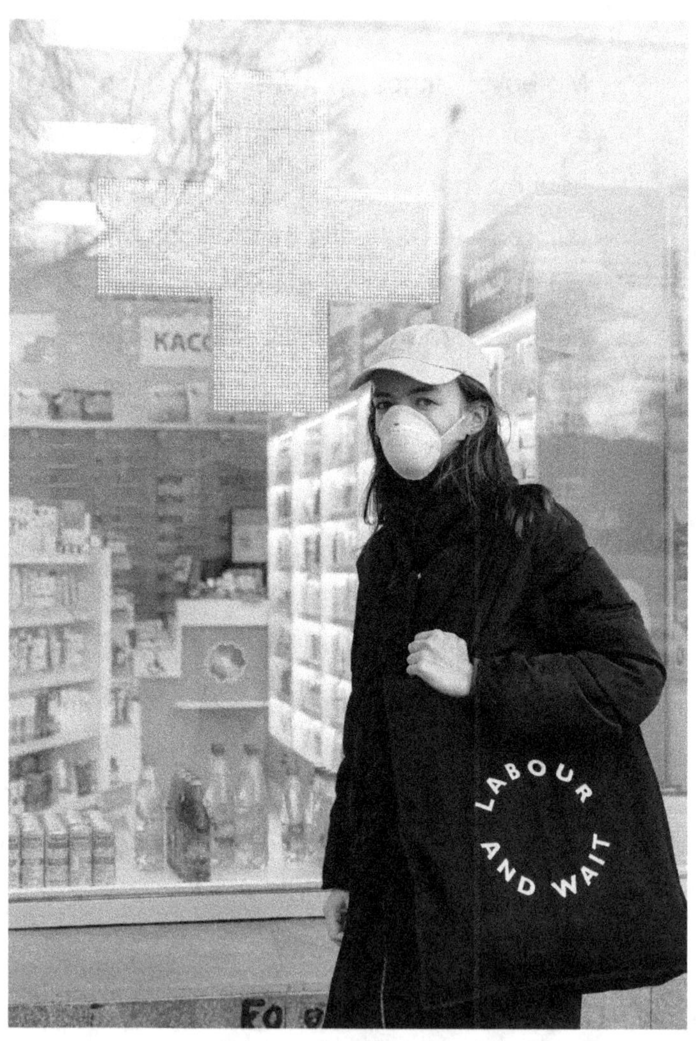

Chapter 5. Medication Management

Medication management plays a pivotal role in the effective control and treatment of various ailments. Proper handling and adherence to prescribed medications are essential for achieving optimal health outcomes. This article explores the significance of medication management in managing different health conditions.

1. Understanding Medication Regimens:
A crucial aspect of medication management involves comprehending prescribed regimens. Patients should be familiar with the names, dosages, and frequencies of their medications. This knowledge empowers individuals to take an active role in their healthcare and ensures they are following the prescribed treatment plan accurately.

2. Adherence to Prescribed Medications:
Consistent adherence to medication schedules is imperative for successful ailment management. Skipping doses or altering the prescribed regimen can compromise the

effectiveness of the treatment. Healthcare providers often emphasize the importance of strict adherence to ensure the desired therapeutic outcomes.

3. Avoiding Medication Interactions:
Medication management also involves being aware of potential interactions between different drugs. Some combinations can lead to adverse effects or diminish the efficacy of certain medications. Patients should communicate openly with their healthcare providers about all the medications, including over-the-counter drugs and supplements, they are currently taking.

4. Monitoring and Reporting Side Effects:
Vigilant monitoring of medication side effects is essential. Patients should be educated on potential adverse reactions and instructed to report any unusual symptoms promptly. This proactive approach allows healthcare providers to adjust medications as needed, ensuring the best possible outcomes while minimizing risks.

5. Communication with Healthcare Providers:
Effective communication between patients and healthcare providers is fundamental in medication management. Regular check-ups and open dialogues enable adjustments to treatment plans based on the patient's response and evolving health conditions.

6. Storage and Disposal:
Proper storage and disposal of medications are often overlooked aspects of medication management. Medications should be stored in accordance with their specific requirements (e.g., temperature, light sensitivity) to maintain their potency. Additionally, safe disposal practices help prevent environmental contamination and accidental ingestion.

Conclusion:
In conclusion, medication management is a critical component of ailment control. Patients who actively engage in understanding their prescribed regimens, adhere to medication schedules, monitor for side effects, and communicate effectively with healthcare providers are more likely to achieve positive health outcomes. By emphasizing the importance of responsible medication management, individuals can take charge of their health and contribute to the success of their treatment plans.

Adhering to Prescribed Medications

Adhering to prescribed medications is crucial for effectively managing ailments. Consistency in taking medications as directed by healthcare professionals helps maintain optimal treatment levels in the body, ensuring the medication's intended effects. Skipping doses or discontinuing treatment prematurely can lead to incomplete recovery, worsened symptoms, or potential complications. It's essential to communicate openly with your healthcare provider about any concerns or challenges related to medication adherence to develop a plan that suits your lifestyle while prioritizing your health.

Understanding Dosages and Side Effects

Understanding dosages and side effects is crucial in effectively managing ailments. Always follow prescribed dosages to ensure the medication's efficacy without risking potential harm. Be vigilant for common side effects such as nausea or drowsiness, but also monitor for rare but serious reactions. Communicate openly with healthcare providers to address concerns and adjust treatment plans if needed, fostering a collaborative approach to wellness.

Chapter 6. Lifestyle Modifications

In the realm of healthcare, lifestyle modification has emerged as a powerful tool for managing various ailments. This proactive approach involves making intentional changes to one's daily habits and behaviors, encompassing aspects like diet, physical activity, sleep, and stress management. Here's a closer look at how lifestyle modification can play a pivotal role in enhancing overall well-being and managing chronic conditions.

1. **Dietary Choices:**
   - Adopting a balanced and nutritious diet is fundamental in managing ailments.
   - Place a focus on lean meats, whole grains, fruits, and vegetables as well as whole meals.
   - Limit intake of processed foods, saturated fats, and excessive sugars.

2. **Physical Activity:**

One of the primary elements of a healthy lifestyle is regular exercise.

- Tailor exercise routines to individual health conditions, focusing on both aerobic and strength training.
- Consult healthcare professionals for personalized exercise plans.

3. **Weight Management**:

- Maintaining a healthy weight is crucial for managing many health conditions.
- Lifestyle changes that promote weight loss, when necessary, can positively impact various ailments, such as diabetes and cardiovascular diseases.

4. **Adequate Sleep:**

- Quality sleep is essential for overall health and healing.

Create a sleep-friendly environment and establish regular sleep schedules.

- Sleep hygiene practices contribute to better management of chronic conditions.

5. **Stress Reduction:**

- Chronic stress can exacerbate ailments; therefore, stress management is vital.
- Include methods of relaxation in everyday activities, such as yoga, deep breathing, or meditation.

- Look for assistance from loved ones, friends, or mental health specialists..

6. Quit Smoking and Limit Alcohol:
- Smoking and excessive alcohol consumption can worsen various health conditions.
- Quitting smoking and moderating alcohol intake contribute significantly to better health outcomes.

7. Regular Health Check-ups:
- Monitoring health regularly aids in early detection and effective management of ailments.
- Schedule routine check-ups and screenings as recommended by healthcare professionals.

8. Educational Resources:
- Continue to learn about your health from reliable sources.
- Engage in health education programs and support groups to enhance understanding and coping mechanisms.

Conclusion:

Embracing lifestyle modification as part of ailment management fosters a holistic and sustainable approach to health. It empowers individuals to take charge of their well-being and complements traditional medical interventions. While each person's journey is unique, the collective impact of positive lifestyle changes contributes to improved outcomes and a better quality of life.

Importance of Healthy Diet

Maintaining a healthy diet is crucial for managing ailments as it provides essential nutrients that support overall well-being. Nutrient-rich foods aid in immune function, help regulate inflammation, and contribute to optimal organ function, assisting the body in coping with various health conditions. Additionally, a balanced diet can help control weight, blood sugar levels, and blood pressure, reducing the risk and severity of chronic diseases. Making informed dietary choices is a proactive step towards enhancing the body's resilience and promoting a better quality of life.

Incorporating Physical Activity

Incorporating physical activity into your routine can be a powerful tool for managing various ailments. Regular exercise can help improve cardiovascular health, reduce inflammation, and enhance overall well-being. For conditions like arthritis, gentle activities like swimming or yoga can alleviate stiffness. Consult with a healthcare professional to tailor a safe and effective exercise plan that suits your specific health needs.

Integrating regular physical activity into your routine can be crucial for managing various ailments. It helps improve cardiovascular health, reduce inflammation, and enhance overall well-being. Consult with a healthcare professional to tailor a suitable exercise plan for your specific condition.

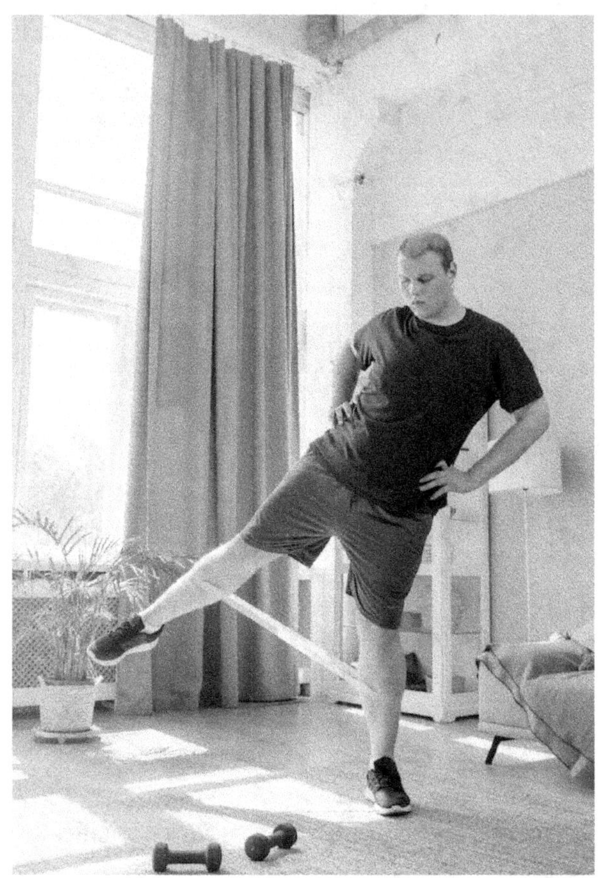

Chapter 7. Stress Management

Stress is a ubiquitous factor in modern life, and its impact on physical and mental health cannot be overstated. The relationship between stress and ailments is well-established, making effective stress management crucial for overall well-being. This comprehensive guide explores the connection between stress and various health conditions, offering practical strategies to manage stress and mitigate its adverse effects on health.

Understanding the Stress-Ailment Connection:

1. **Physiological Impact:**
   - Chronic stress triggers the release of stress hormones like cortisol, which, when prolonged, can lead to inflammation and weaken the immune system.
   - Elevated stress levels are linked to cardiovascular issues, compromised digestive health, and disruptions in sleep patterns.

2. Mental Health Consequences:

- Stress is a significant contributor to mental health disorders such as anxiety and depression.
- Chronic stress can exacerbate existing conditions and hinder the recovery process.

Effective Stress Management Strategies:

1. Mindfulness and Meditation:

- Incorporating mindfulness practices, like meditation and deep breathing exercises, can calm the mind and reduce stress.
- Mindfulness helps individuals stay present, fostering a sense of control over their thoughts and emotions.

2. Physical Activity:

- Regular exercise releases endorphins, the body's natural mood enhancers, helping to alleviate stress.
- Engaging in physical activity also promotes better sleep, which is crucial for overall health.

3. Healthy Lifestyle Choices:

- Prioritizing a balanced diet with nutrient-rich foods supports the body's resilience to stress.

- Adequate hydration and limiting the intake of stimulants like caffeine and alcohol contribute to overall well-being.

4. Establishing Support Systems:
- Building a strong social support network provides avenues for sharing concerns and receiving emotional support.
- Open communication with friends, family, or mental health professionals can be pivotal in stress management.

5. Time Management:
- Efficiently organizing and prioritizing tasks helps prevent feelings of overwhelm.
- Setting realistic goals and breaking them down into manageable steps fosters a sense of accomplishment.

6. Cognitive Behavioral Therapy (CBT):
- CBT is an evidence-based therapeutic approach that helps individuals identify and change negative thought patterns contributing to stress.
- Learning coping mechanisms through CBT can enhance resilience and reduce the impact of stress on ailments.

Integrating Stress Management into Daily Life:

1. **Routine Check-ins:**
   - Regularly assess stress levels and adjust management strategies accordingly.
   - Consistency in stress management practices is key for long-term benefits.

2. **Holistic Approaches:**
   - Combining multiple stress management techniques enhances their effectiveness.
   - Addressing the root causes of stress while implementing coping strategies provides a more comprehensive approach.

In conclusion, stress management plays a pivotal role in managing ailments. By adopting a holistic approach that encompasses physical, mental, and lifestyle factors, individuals can empower themselves to mitigate the impact of stress on their overall health. Consistent effort towards stress reduction not only promotes well-being but also contributes to the prevention and management of various health conditions.

Identifying and Coping with Stressors

Identifying and coping with stressors in managing ailments requires a comprehensive approach. Start by recognizing potential stressors, such as treatment challenges, lifestyle adjustments, and emotional concerns. Develop coping strategies like mindfulness, relaxation techniques, and seeking social support. Communication with healthcare professionals, maintaining a healthy routine, and staying informed about your condition also play crucial roles in effective stress management during the journey of managing ailments.

Relaxation Techniques

Certainly! Relaxation techniques can be beneficial for managing various ailments. Here are some techniques to consider:

1. **Deep Breathing**: Practice diaphragmatic breathing to calm the nervous system and reduce stress. Exhale slowly through your lips

after taking a big breath through your nose and contracting your abdomen.

2. **Progressive Muscle Relaxation (PMR):** Tense and then release different muscle groups to promote physical relaxation. Work your way up to your head starting at your toes.

3. **Mindfulness Meditation:** Focus on the present moment without judgment. Mindfulness can help alleviate symptoms associated with chronic pain, anxiety, and depression.

4. **Guided Imagery:** Visualize peaceful scenes or positive outcomes. This can shift your focus away from pain or discomfort, promoting a sense of calm.

5. **Yoga:** Gentle yoga poses and stretches can improve flexibility, reduce tension, and enhance overall well-being. Choose poses suitable for your physical condition.

6. **Tai Chi:** This gentle martial art involves slow, flowing movements that can improve balance,

flexibility, and relaxation. It's particularly beneficial for arthritis and chronic pain.

7. **Autogenic Training**: A self-help relaxation technique involving visualizing and verbalizing sensations of warmth and heaviness to promote relaxation.

8. **Aromatherapy**: Use calming scents like lavender or chamomile to create a soothing environment. Essential oils can be diffused or applied topically (after proper dilution).

9. **Hot Baths or Showers**: Warm water can relax muscles and alleviate tension. Add Epsom salts to the bath for added benefits.

10. **Biofeedback:** This technique involves monitoring and controlling physiological functions, such as heart rate and muscle tension, to promote relaxation.

Always consult with healthcare professionals before trying new relaxation techniques,

especially if you have pre-existing medical
conditions. These practices can complement
medical treatments but should not replace
professional advice.

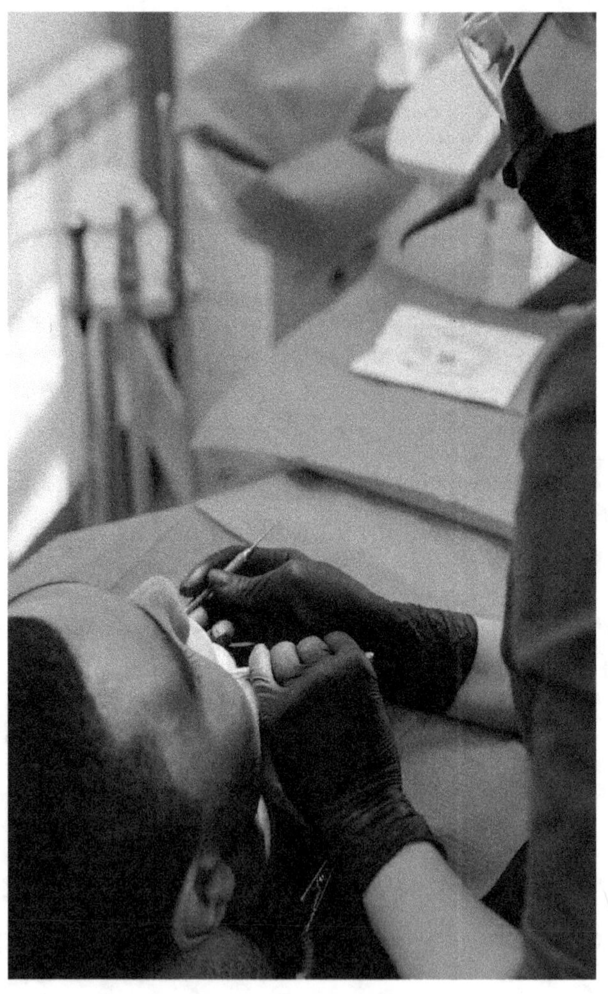

Chapter 8. Support Systems

Support systems play a crucial role in effectively managing ailments, providing individuals with the necessary tools and assistance to cope with the physical, emotional, and psychological challenges associated with various health conditions. These support systems encompass a wide range of elements, including healthcare professionals, family and friends, community resources, and technological aids.

1. **Healthcare Professionals:**
    - **Physicians and Specialists:** Primary care physicians and specialists contribute to ailment management through diagnosis, treatment plans, and ongoing medical supervision.
    - **Nurses and Caregivers:** These professionals offer essential support in administering treatments, monitoring symptoms, and providing emotional care.

2. **Family and Friends:**
   - **Emotional Support:** The emotional backing from loved ones can significantly impact an individual's mental well-being during the ailment management process.
   - **Practical Assistance:** Family and friends often play a key role in providing practical help, such as transportation to medical appointments or assistance with daily activities.

3. **Community Resources:**
   - **Support Groups:** Joining support groups allows individuals with similar ailments to share experiences, advice, and emotional support, fostering a sense of community.
   - **Nonprofit Organizations:** These organizations often provide valuable resources, information, and financial assistance for individuals managing specific ailments.

4. **Technology and Innovations:**
   - **Telemedicine:** Remote consultations and monitoring tools enable individuals to connect with healthcare professionals conveniently, especially useful for those with chronic conditions.
   - **Health Apps and Wearables:** Mobile applications and wearable devices help

individuals track and manage their health, providing real-time data to both patients and healthcare providers.

5. **Educational Resources:**
   - **Health Literacy Programs:** Educational initiatives empower individuals to understand their ailments better, promoting informed decision-making and self-management.
   - **Online Information:** Access to reliable online resources helps individuals stay informed about their condition, treatment options, and potential lifestyle modifications.

6. **Psychological Support:**
   - **Therapists and Counselors:** Mental health professionals assist individuals in coping with the emotional and psychological impact of their ailments.
   - **Mindfulness and Relaxation Techniques:** Techniques such as meditation and mindfulness can be effective in reducing stress and improving overall well-being.

7. **Financial Support:**
   - **Insurance Programs:** Adequate insurance coverage ensures that individuals have access to necessary

medical treatments without facing significant financial burdens.

- **Government Assistance:** Some individuals may qualify for government assistance programs that provide financial support for medical expenses.

In conclusion, a comprehensive support system that combines medical expertise, emotional support from family and friends, community resources, technological innovations, educational tools, psychological assistance, and financial support is essential for effectively managing ailments. This holistic approach addresses the diverse needs of individuals, enhancing their overall well-being and resilience in the face of health challenges.

Building a Supportive Network

Living with ailments can be challenging, both physically and emotionally. Building a supportive network is crucial for effectively managing health conditions. In this guide, we explore the importance of a supportive network and provide practical tips for creating and maintaining one.

1. **Family and Friends:**
   - Communicate openly with your close circle about your health condition.
   - Educate them on your needs and how they can offer support.
   - Encourage honest conversations to strengthen emotional bonds.

2. **Healthcare Professionals:**
   - Foster a collaborative relationship with your healthcare team.
   - Regularly communicate your concerns, progress, and any changes in your condition.
   - Seek guidance on building a holistic health management plan.

3. **Online Communities:**
   - Join online forums or social media groups related to your ailment.
   - Share experiences, advice, and learn from others facing similar challenges.
   - Be cautious of misinformation and focus on reputable sources.

4. **Support Groups:**
   - Attend local support groups for your specific ailment.
   - Connect with individuals who understand the daily struggles you face.
   - Community building and the sharing of coping mechanisms are encouraged.

5. **Educate Your Network**:
- Provide information about your ailment to friends and family.
- Help them understand the impact on your life and the support you may require.
- Knowledge reduces stigma and fosters empathy.

6. **Empower Others to Help:**
- Clearly express how friends and family can assist you.
- Assign specific tasks based on your needs, making it easier for them to help.
- Appreciate and acknowledge their support regularly.

7. **Self-Care Support**:
- Prioritize self-care to better manage your health.
- Communicate your self-care routines and enlist support when needed.
- Encourage loved ones to engage in self-care practices as well.

8. **Celebrate Achievements:**
- Acknowledge and celebrate milestones in your health journey.
- Share achievements with your support network to reinforce positivity.
- Create a culture of encouragement and resilience.

9. **Open Lines of Communication**:
- Establish clear communication channels within your network.
- Keep loved ones informed about changes in your health status.
- Regularly check in with your support system.

Conclusion:
Building a supportive network is an essential aspect of effectively managing ailments. By cultivating open communication, educating those around you, and actively engaging with various support channels, you can create a robust network that contributes to your overall well-being. Remember, you're not alone in your journey, and a strong support system can make a significant difference in your health and quality of life.

Joining Support Groups

Joining support groups can be invaluable in managing ailments. These groups provide a sense of community, understanding, and shared experiences, which can offer emotional support. Additionally, members often share valuable information about coping strategies, treatment options, and lifestyle adjustments. Connecting with others facing similar challenges can foster a sense of belonging and empowerment, ultimately enhancing the overall well-being of individuals managing ailments

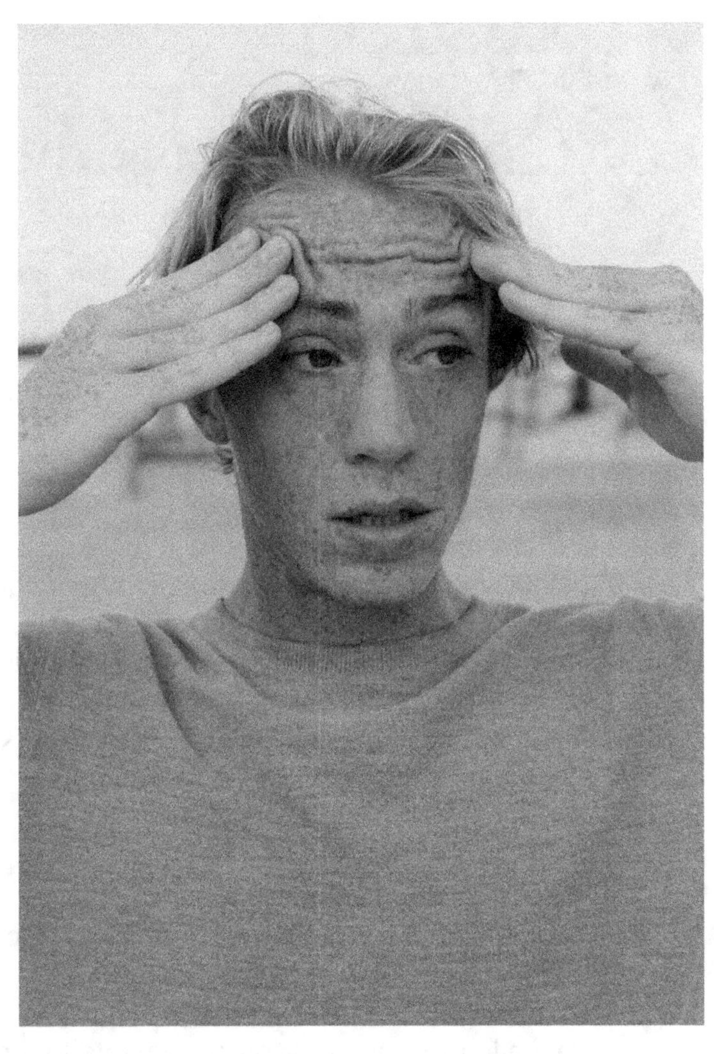

Chapter 9. Preventive Measures

Preventive Measures for Managing Ailments

Preventive measures play a crucial role in maintaining overall well-being and managing various ailments. By adopting proactive strategies, individuals can significantly reduce the risk of developing health issues and enhance their quality of life. Here are key preventive measures that contribute to effectively managing ailments.

1. **Regular Health Check-ups:**
Scheduling routine health check-ups allows early detection of potential health issues. Timely identification enables prompt intervention, preventing the progression of ailments to more severe stages.

2. **Healthy Lifestyle Choices:**
Adopting a balanced and nutritious diet, engaging in regular physical activity, and avoiding harmful habits like smoking and

excessive alcohol consumption contribute to overall health. These lifestyle choices help prevent a range of ailments, including cardiovascular diseases and obesity.

3. **Stress Management:**

Chronic stress can adversely impact health, contributing to various ailments. Incorporating stress management techniques such as mindfulness, meditation, and relaxation exercises promotes mental well-being and aids in preventing stress-related health issues.

4. **Immunization**:

Keeping vaccinations up-to-date is a crucial preventive measure. Immunizations protect against various infectious diseases, reducing the likelihood of contracting illnesses and preventing the spread of contagious conditions within communities.

5. **Proper Hygiene Practices:**

Simple hygiene habits, such as regular handwashing, proper dental care, and maintaining cleanliness in living spaces, play a pivotal role in preventing the spread of infections and minimizing the risk of ailments.

6. **Adequate Sleep:**

Quality sleep is essential for overall health and well-being. Establishing a consistent sleep routine helps the body recover and strengthens the immune system, reducing susceptibility to various health issues.

7. **Regular Exercise:**

Physical activity not only helps in maintaining a healthy weight but also boosts cardiovascular health, improves mood, and enhances overall fitness. Regular exercise is a fundamental preventive measure for managing ailments like diabetes, hypertension, and musculoskeletal disorders.

8. **Screen Time Management:**

Excessive screen time, especially on digital devices, can contribute to various health issues, including eye strain and disrupted sleep patterns. Setting limits on screen time and incorporating breaks are essential for preventing associated ailments.

9. **Awareness and Education:**

Staying informed about potential health risks, understanding family medical history, and educating oneself about preventive measures empower individuals to make informed decisions about their health.

10. **Maintaining a Supportive Social Network:**

Strong social connections positively impact mental and emotional well-being. Building and maintaining a supportive social network can contribute to stress reduction and provide assistance during challenging times.

Conclusion:

Preventive measures are a cornerstone in the management of ailments, offering a proactive approach to maintaining health and preventing the onset of various conditions. By incorporating these strategies into daily life, individuals can take significant steps towards a healthier and more resilient future.

Immunizations and Vaccinations

Immunization and vaccinations play a crucial role in managing and preventing a wide range of ailments. These medical interventions stimulate the immune system to recognize and combat specific pathogens, such as bacteria or viruses, reducing the risk of infections and their associated complications.

One of the primary benefits of immunization is the prevention of contagious diseases. Vaccines have been instrumental in eradicating or controlling numerous infectious diseases, like polio, measles, and smallpox. This not only protects individuals but also contributes to the overall public health by creating herd immunity, making it more challenging for diseases to spread within communities.

Vaccines are particularly vital in safeguarding vulnerable populations, including infants, elderly individuals, and those with weakened immune systems. By providing a shield against diseases, vaccines help prevent severe illnesses, hospitalizations, and potential long-term complications.

In addition to their role in infectious disease prevention, vaccines also contribute to managing the burden on healthcare systems. By reducing the incidence of preventable diseases, vaccinations alleviate the strain on medical resources and minimize the economic impact associated with treating and containing outbreaks.

Continuous research and development in the field of immunization have led to the creation of vaccines for emerging threats, such as novel viruses. This adaptability is crucial in addressing evolving health challenges and maintaining preparedness against potential pandemics.

It's essential for individuals to stay informed about recommended vaccination schedules and ensure that they and their communities are adequately protected. Public awareness campaigns and healthcare initiatives play a pivotal role in promoting vaccine acceptance and countering misinformation.

In conclusion, immunization and vaccinations serve as powerful tools in managing ailments by preventing the onset and spread of infectious diseases. As ongoing advancements in medical science continue, vaccines remain a cornerstone of public health strategies, offering protection, promoting well-being, and contributing to the overall resilience of global healthcare systems.

Regular Health Screenings

Regular health screenings play a crucial role in managing ailments by detecting potential issues early on. Screenings, such as blood pressure checks, cholesterol tests, and cancer screenings, help identify risk factors and allow for timely intervention. This proactive approach enables healthcare professionals to initiate preventive measures, reducing the impact and severity of ailments. Consistent screenings contribute to overall well-being and can be instrumental in maintaining a healthy lifestyle.

Chapter 10. Emergency Preparedness

A Guide to Emergency Preparedness: Managing Ailments with Confidence

In times of crisis, being well-prepared for emergencies can make a significant difference, especially when it comes to managing ailments. Whether it's a natural disaster, power outage, or unforeseen circumstances, having a plan in place ensures you can address health concerns effectively. Here's a comprehensive guide to help you navigate emergency preparedness in managing ailments:

1. Create a Medical Emergency Kit:

- Assemble a well-stocked first aid kit with essential supplies such as bandages, antiseptic wipes, pain relievers, and any prescribed medications.
- Ensure your kit is easily accessible and periodically check its contents for expiration dates.

2. Maintain a Personal Health Record:

- Keep a detailed record of your medical history, including current medications, allergies, and any pre-existing conditions.
- Include emergency contacts and healthcare providers in your record.

3. Communication Plan:

- Establish a communication strategy with family, friends, and healthcare providers in case of emergencies.
- Share your medical information with trusted individuals who can assist you during a crisis.

4. Stay Informed:

- Know the common health risks associated with your geographical location and prepare accordingly.
- Stay updated on local emergency procedures and evacuation routes.

5. Power Outage Preparedness:

- If you rely on electronic medical devices, have backup power sources like portable chargers or generators.
- Keep a supply of medications that do not require refrigeration.

6. Emergency Evacuation Plan:

- Develop a plan for evacuating your home if necessary. Consider mobility challenges and plan for assistance if needed.
- Ensure you have a portable bag with necessary medical supplies for a quick departure.

7. Community Resources:

- Identify local emergency shelters and healthcare facilities in your area.
- Connect with community support groups for individuals with similar health concerns.

8. Regular Health Check-ups:

- Schedule routine health check-ups to monitor and manage your ailments effectively.
- Discuss emergency preparedness with your healthcare provider for personalized advice.

9. Medication Management:

- Keep an adequate supply of prescription medications on hand.
- Rotate medications to prevent expiration, and consider automatic prescription refills where available.

10. Educate Family and Caregivers:

- Ensure that family members, friends, or caregivers are familiar with your emergency plan and know how to assist you during health crises.

By proactively addressing emergency preparedness in managing ailments, you empower yourself to face unexpected situations confidently. Remember to adapt these guidelines to your specific health needs and consult with healthcare professionals for personalized advice. Stay vigilant, stay prepared, and prioritize your well-being in all circumstances.

Creating an Emergency Plan

Creating an emergency plan for managing ailments involves several key steps. Firstly, identify the specific ailment and understand its symptoms and triggers. Develop a list of emergency contacts, including healthcare professionals and family members.

Next, outline a step-by-step response plan, detailing actions to take during an emergency. Include information on medication administration, if applicable, and note any allergies or sensitivities. Ensure that all relevant medical records and documents are easily accessible.

Regularly review and update the emergency plan to reflect any changes in the ailment, medications, or contact information. Additionally, share the plan with trusted individuals who may need to assist in case of an emergency. Practicing the plan through simulations can help ensure everyone involved is familiar with the necessary procedures.

Knowing When to Seek Urgent Care

Knowing when to seek urgent care is crucial in managing ailments. If you experience severe pain, difficulty breathing, sudden weakness, or signs of a serious infection, it's advisable to seek immediate medical attention. Trust your instincts and prioritize urgent care for symptoms that could indicate a life-threatening situation. If in doubt, it's always better to err on the side of caution and seek prompt medical assistance.

Chapter 11. Conclusion

Managing ailments involves a holistic approach that combines medical treatment, lifestyle adjustments, and emotional well-being. Obtain advice from medical specialists for precise diagnosis and individualized treatment programs.Adopt a balanced diet, engage in regular exercise, and prioritize sufficient sleep to support overall health. Stay informed about your condition, follow prescribed medications, and attend regular check-ups. Manage stress through relaxation techniques and seek emotional support when needed. Embrace a positive mindset, as mental health plays a crucial role in overall well-being. Remember, effective ailment management is a collaborative effort between you, your healthcare team, and a healthy lifestyle.

Recap of Ailment Management Strategies

Managing ailments effectively involves a multifaceted approach that encompasses various strategies. From lifestyle modifications to medical interventions, a comprehensive plan is essential. Let's recap some key ailment management strategies:

1. **Healthy Lifestyle Habits:**
   - **Dietary Changes:** Emphasize a balanced diet with an emphasis on fruits, vegetables, and whole grains. Limiting processed foods and reducing salt intake can be beneficial.
   - **Regular Exercise:** Physical activity contributes to overall well-being. Tailor exercise routines to individual abilities and medical conditions.

2. **Medication Adherence:**
   - **Consistent Medication Use:** Follow prescribed medication schedules diligently. Missing doses or discontinuing medications without consulting a healthcare professional can hinder progress.

3. **Stress Management:**
   - **Mind-Body Techniques:** Practices such as meditation, deep breathing exercises, and yoga can help manage stress, which is often linked to various ailments.

4. **Regular Medical Check-ups:**
   - **Monitoring and Adjusting Treatment Plans:** Regular visits to healthcare

providers allow for monitoring the ailment's progression. Adjustments to treatment plans can be made based on individual responses.

5. Educational Resources:

- **Patient Education:** Understanding the ailment, its triggers, and management options empowers individuals to actively participate in their care.

6. Support Systems:

- **Family and Community Support:** Having a strong support system can significantly impact mental and emotional well-being, providing encouragement and assistance when needed.

7. Holistic Approaches:

- **Complementary Therapies:** Some individuals find relief through complementary therapies like acupuncture, massage, or herbal remedies.

It is imperative, therefore, that medical specialists be consulted prior to implementing these in a therapeutic regimen.

8. Technology Integration:

- **Health Apps and Wearables:** Utilize technology to track symptoms, medications, and vital signs. This information can be shared with healthcare providers for better-informed decisions.

9. **Self-Monitoring:**
   - **Symptom Tracking:** Regularly monitoring symptoms and noting any changes helps in identifying patterns and potential triggers, aiding in proactive management.

10. **Collaborative Care:**
   - **Multidisciplinary Approach:** Coordinated care involving various healthcare professionals ensures a holistic view of the ailment, addressing both physical and psychological aspects.

Remember, effective ailment management is often an ongoing process that requires commitment and collaboration between individuals, healthcare providers, and support networks. Always consult with healthcare professionals for personalized advice based on specific conditions.

Encouragement for Continued Well-being

Taking care of your well-being while managing ailments is crucial. Keep in mind that even though development is slow, every little step matters. Surround yourself with a supportive network, stay informed about your condition, and focus on positive lifestyle changes. Celebrate your victories, no matter how small, and prioritize self-care to enhance your overall well-being.